Letters to My Bipolar Self

A representation of powerful acts of self-love to mentally heal myself and to empower others to incorporate self-love unapologetically

Volume 1

Letters to My Bipolar Self

Letters to My Bipolar Self

Letters to My Bipolar Self

Volume 1

written and created by
Glenda Lezeau

Letters to My Bipolar Self

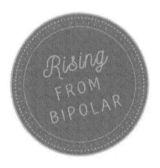

Book Cover design by Opeyemi (@crea8tive on Fiverr.com)
Book Cover photography by Meange Adeclat
Front and Back Cover Photography edited by
Meange Adeclat and Sehvrine Lezeau
ISBN 978-1-7341888-0-6 (paperback)
Manuscript edited by AnJu Hyppolite and Wynnie Lamour
Interior formatting by BlackGold Publishing
Back cover edited by Wynnie Lamour and Janice Lezeau
Published by Water Wave Press www.risingfrombipolar.com

DISCLAIMER

I hope you find this book helpful and empowering, but this book is not meant to substitute medical and/or psychological treatment. I am not a certified mental health professional, so everything that I mention in this book is based on my personal experiences. Please do not use this book as a replacement of therapy or psychological services, especially if you are experiencing unbearable symptoms or you are in the middle of a mental health crisis.

Having suicidal thoughts?

Call 1-800-273-8255 (National Suicide Prevention Line; 24/7) and ask for support from a friend, loved one, or mental health professional.

Having any type of mental health crisis?

Text: 741741 (Crisis Text Line; 24/7)

Letters to My Bipolar Self

Letters to My Bipolar Self

I dedicate this book...

to my sister, Janice,
who I am convinced was born with special skills that
help me when I'm experiencing symptoms. You
always know how to handle me in the best way in
those moments, even when no one else knows what
is happening to me! Thank you for ALWAYS being
there when I need you the most. I love you beyond
words and could not have asked for a better sister.

to my parents who support me left, right, and all
around: THANK YOU SOOOOO much for all that you
do for me and my condition. You give me a reason to
fight through the pain and push through my
symptoms. I am not sure how I would survive
without you. I feel like my symptoms would be a lot
worse if I did not have the two of you to help me
through them. I truly love you so much!

to my Grandma and my WHOLE Lezeau family —
I am grateful for you. And also, no matter what
anyone says, follow what you feel destined to do as
long as it is positive. Keep in mind what this book
symbolizes... Lezeau Book or No Book
(haha *inside joke*) Love ya!

to those who visited me whenever I was admitted to
the psychiatric unit: You have seen me at my worst,
but continue to be there for me. Special thanks to my
Dad for coming twice a day, for my Mom coming
every day after work, and for my sister who traveled
miles to see me. Thank you so much.

Letters to My Bipolar Self

to my editor, AnJu,
who is also my accountability partner in
EVERYTHING and continuously supports me in a
variety of ways! Thank you for being present with me
and pushing me to get work done on a weekly basis!!

to my editor and very dear friend Wynnie
who is ALWAYS ready to support or help me in any
way possible. You push me past my fears and
continuously remind me of my worth. Thank you for
constantly proving to me that you are there for me
whenever I need you. You will always hold a special
place in my heart!

to Jean from ACA Branding Agency:
Thank you for your guidance in the beginning stages
and for making my vision better than what I could
ever visualized!

to Helyn from Talentpreneurship Academy and
Helyn's corner: I am convinced that meeting you was
divinely connected. Thank you so much for your
book writing workshop and for your AMAZING
advice on the pre-launch process. You were so
patient in guiding me! You are a great part of any
success that comes from this book!

to all who have supported me with my condition:
I appreciate every little moment of support.

Letters to My Bipolar Self

to all those who have heard my story and chose to support me rather than judge me.

to all the amazing clinicians who have positively impacted me and didn't make me feel like just another patient.

to my first therapist and current therapist – the two of you have dramatically changed my life. I am forever grateful for you. Thank you for all that you have done for me! Special shoutout to my current therapist who has gotten me through the worst of times and continues to guide me in my healing practices. You are very relatable, and it is so cool that we have a lot in common.

to my awesome, amazing, dope, comical friends and supporters: I truly love each and every one of you. I am blessed to have you.

Special Thanks…

This book could not have been published without the help of these amazing, talented individuals. Thank you, thank you, and *thank you!*

Meange Adeclat (Photography)
AnJu Hyppolite (Editor)
Wynnie Lamour-Quansah (Editor)
Sehvrine Lezeau (Edited Photos)
BlackGold Publishing (Interior Formatting)

I would also like to acknowledge and list the first 8 people who bought my book during pre-sales. Special thanks to all of you! Your support is noticed and sincerely appreciated. You have blessed me and in return I hope you will receive many blessings your way.

Quiana V.

Brittany Ro

Lhomel C.

Suky L.

Tashelle L.

Janice L.

Mom

Dad

Thank you all so much.

My Beloved Readers,

First and foremost, my appreciation for you is tremendous! Thank you for reading my truth as I share my journey with bipolar disorder. I was diagnosed in 2011 and was inspired to help others through my story. My story is not just for those with bipolar disorder or those with a mental health condition. It is meant to educate and empower anyone and everyone.

I mostly wrote these 50 letters to myself in real time. If I did not complete the letters on the date you see on them, I at least wrote down the concept on that date and then wrote the letter, in full, at a later date. In the letters, I use terms of endearment to show self-affection and self-love despite my condition. I have written all of the letters to myself, even the ones that are signed *Your Secret Admirer*. I hope that these letters inspire the growing relationship that you have with yourself. After all, it is one of the most important relationships and helps guide you into doing what's best for you. Feel free to re-write any of these letters to yourself and personalize it in any way you want to. These letters are also ideal to read during moments of depression or anxiety when you don't feel like doing much to overcome those moments. Reading a letter is something simple that I like to implement as part of my wellness regime and you can do the same. I know it may seem a little weird at first to read or write these letters to yourself. Once you understand the concept and start doing it, it is very therapeutic. You can even become emotional from writing some letters if you dig deep. Keep an open mindset. Writing these letters and re-reading them over time has been very therapeutic for me.

Oh, and I am a proud Haitian, so you will notice some words in Haitian Creole with the English translation at the bottom.

Yours Truly,

Glenda

Letters to My Bipolar Self

Table of Contents

Letters to My Bipolar Self

#1

A Beautiful Transformation

10/2/2016

"The past reveals dark times as if it represents a flower in the winter, but now you have blossomed since the seasons have changed to spring."

My Dearest Love,

Always remember how beautiful you are inside and out. I am beyond proud of who you are and who you've become. The past reveals dark times as if it represents a flower in the winter, but now you have blossomed since the seasons have changed to spring. The confidence and positivity that you have developed are admirable. I know you will accomplish all that you want, but be in the present and embrace the process. And of course...PRAY, PRAY, PRAY! Stay humble and keep blossoming. Love you, Boo.

Your biggest fan,

Glenda

Letters to My Bipolar Self

Write notes or your own letter:

#2

Mental Breakdown

12/22/2016

"I see your mental breakdown as a release of stress and the need to re-shift some things."

My Sweetheart,

My heart hurts from what you went through yesterday. It's been five years since you had your first and only mental breakdown, but yesterday you had your second. I know this is shocking to you because you thought that you would never have another one again, but it happened. It's good to see that you are starting to feel better though!

Even though you relapsed after five years, take a look at how far you have come! The manic phase didn't even last that long. It only lasted for about an hour or so. Five years ago, it lasted on and off for a whole week! You also did an amazing job of recognizing your symptoms right away and immediately getting the help that you needed. And because of that, your symptoms did not escalate into having you admitted into the hospital. Wow!! I am amazed at how much you've changed and grown mentally. You are so much stronger mentally that you escaped hospitalization. My favorite part was when you were talking on the phone to your sister so that she could keep you calm, and in the middle of your manic phase you would tell her, "I'm going to be fine. I will not end up in the hospital this time." You were speaking affirmations out loud several times. Remember those moments when you think you failed for having a relapse.

I see your mental breakdown as a release of stress and the need to re-shift some things. I know you feel the same way since you started jotting down several "re-shifts" that you need to do. Refer back to that list as you are on the road to recovery. Give yourself time to heal. You will get through this and will become stronger than ever!

I wish you a speedy and amazing recovery!

Kisses and hugs,

You Know Who

#3

Depressive Mood Dissolves in Seconds

3/24/17

"Remember this moment."

Hey Love|

Remember this moment. Remember the moment when your depressive mood from last night lingered on into today and was switched off in a matter of seconds. It wasn't even intentional. The Universe just made some alignments knowing what would make you smile and laugh. One smile. One giggle. And just like that, you were better!

Remember this moment...

So that you can remind yourself of the moment you overcame a depressive state. So that you can uplift yourself the next time you feel like giving up or the next time it feels like the depressive state will last forever.

Keep rising and keep shining.

XOXO

Your Secret Admirer

Letters to My Bipolar Self

Write notes or your own letter:

#4

Depression with No Strength

4/1/17

"Your strength and courage are just temporarily disabled."

Hey Boo,

Just know...

When you feel like giving up, when you are drowning in tears, when you have no strength...

Know that some of it is a lie. You do have strength but just in the moment, it seems as if you don't. Your strength and courage are just temporarily disabled. Tell yourself that and rationalize those thoughts. Think of an alternative to the problem instead of thinking the problem has defeated you. Don't lead yourself down a downward spiral banister by thinking of all the ways that you can't do something. Instead, walk yourself up the stairs one step at a time thinking of alternative ways that you can achieve that thing that you want to give up on and getting back that strength you thought you lost. If it feels too challenging to do on your own, just know that you are not alone. Ask God to either help you or send someone or something your way to help you up the stairs. You never know what unexpected assistance will make it easier to climb the stairs, so keep an open heart and welcome him, her, or it with open arms.

Here's me opening my arms to you for a big hug!

~You know who :)

Letters to My Bipolar Self

Write notes or your own letter:

#5

It Can Happen

4/2/17

"When irrational thoughts
crush your dreams, just
know... it can happen."

My Dreamer,

Today you heard a message titled,
It can happen. The title alone says a lot.

When irrational thoughts crush your dreams, just know... it can happen.

When you feel like giving up, just know...

it can happen.

When you have already given up, just know...

it can happen.

Continue to be my favorite little dreamer.

Your wish is my command,

G. Nee

Letters to My Bipolar Self

Write notes or your own letter:

#6

Practice Gratitude

4/13/17

"Applaud yourself for even the smallest progress that you have made."

Hey My Love!

So, I noticed that you practice gratitude continuously but you need to do it more aggressively. There are times where you still can't help but to be not as grateful as you should be. I don't think it's because you're an ungrateful being. I think you don't feel as grateful when anxiety strikes...when your anxiety reminds you that you are not where you thought you should be by now or haven't reached certain goals yet. Try your best to be present. Applaud yourself for even the smallest progress that you have made. And while you are on your way to reaching for the stars through the sky, be extremely grateful for ALL that you have in the present. Whenever your anxiety hits and leads you to having a bout of ungratefulness, keep pushing yourself to shift your focus to ALL that you should be grateful for.

I know for one that I'm grateful for you; you just being you.

Love you.

By: You know who.

Letters to My Bipolar Self

Write notes or your own letter:

#7

No Energy To Pursue Visions

4/26/17

"Whenever you feel this way, you just need to find a strand of motivation to continue."

Hola!

Your visions and goals are very powerful! You are very ambitious, but sometimes you don't feel energized to pursue your visions. Whenever you feel this way, you just need to find a strand of motivation to continue. The path that you are on is not a "normal" path, so it is easy to beat yourself up for choosing not to walk down a "normal" path. Don't beat yourself up. You are entitled to have visions and will reach a part of the path where your vision becomes your reality. I know that the current part of the path that you are on is causing you to have anxiety and depressive states. Some of these states are caused by all the different jobs that you have had. You have been job hopping for a while now. I know it is frustrating, but your dissatisfaction in all these jobs that you have had is proof that you need to focus on pursuing your visions. Use your job hopping to energize you to continue to walk on your path of your visions and goals. The path is curvy with lots of steep hills. The more you exercise while on this path, the stronger you will be to handle the rest of the path.

Keep walking,

Your Coach

Letters to My Bipolar Self

Write notes or your own letter:

#8

Joy

4/27/17

"Believe that it is already within you, deep inside your depression."

Hey you!

Let's talk...

about joy;

about when joy seems nonexistent;

about its existence even when you don't see it.

Believe that it is already within you, deep inside your depression. Believe that it will find you again...in a familiar or foreign form. I promise it will. Because it just happened to you. After weeks of feeling that joy was nonexistent, you just felt moments of joy and excitement when seeing certain visions come to play and meeting with people that you love. Joy found you again and it will continue to find you again...and again.

I'm filled with joy! And so are you!

Joyfully,

Glenda

Letters to My Bipolar Self

Write notes or your own letter:

#9

Feeling Depressed

4/28/17

"Just don't believe the irrational thinking around those topics."

My Love,

Are you feeling depressed? If so, know that during this moment a lot of the thoughts that are running through your mind are lies. You are thinking of thoughts and accusations that are false. Do your best to dismiss those thoughts, especially the ones that don't normally sound like you or ones that contradict what you truly believe. But at the same time, take some mental notes on the topics that are on your mind because that could give you an idea of what changes you might need to make. Just don't believe the irrational thinking around those topics.

I know it's traumatizing to experience this moment, but keep reassuring yourself that this too shall pass and that you are strong enough to conquer it. On the bright side, there is always something that you can learn from depressive moments. While you are feeling depressed, validate your feelings, empathize with yourself, be patient with yourself, and be forgiving to yourself.

I love you, even when you are in this state.

XOXO,

Your cheerleader

Letters to My Bipolar Self

Write notes or your own letter:

#10

One Job After the Next..
and the Next...

5/2/17

"I am not judging you at all!
So, don't judge yourself
either."

Hello There‼

How are you? Wait, don't answer that. I already know. :) I've been reflecting on something that seems to be a recurring cycle for you: job experiences. It seems to be getting out of control with the amount of jobs you keep quitting because of negative experiences or realizations the job is not a good fit for you. Teaching Kreyòl seems to be the only job that you genuinely enjoy and have done consistently, but it is more of a freelance position. Other than that (and the mailroom job in college), you haven't liked ANY job that you've done. You have done jobs in almost every industry with various environments and still have not found a good match. I am not judging you at all! So, don't judge yourself either. I know it is frustrating that you keep trying different positions and getting the same results. I do not have the complete answer as to why. Some people might think it's because of your condition and I don't know if that has something to do with it, but I honestly feel deep inside that this cycle keeps happening because you are meant to work for yourself to create your own projects. Don't give up because you are frustrated at being in the same situation over and over again with different jobs. Don't feel embarrassed because people are judging you based on all the jobs that you have had and have left. As much as you feel like a failure every time you start a job that you thought you would have liked and realize that you really don't, use it as a lesson. Applaud yourself for your bravery in not

39

settling at a job simply because of "good benefits". Also, remember that even when you are at a job that you don't belong in, God still finds an opportunity to work in you while you are there. There have been situations where you met people at work who you knew were God-sent or you learned certain skills at one job that were unexpectedly transferable to the next job. So, no matter what, God is still with you even at a job where you do not fit in. Use these negative experiences as a guiding force to persistently and continuously work towards your personal goals and dreams. Make the time to diligently work on your creative projects on the side so that eventually your projects will become successful and you will not have to worry about having to do a job you don't belong at or quitting yet another job.

Keep your head above water and find ways to continuously re-motivate yourself in the process to your own successes. I truly believe in you and your amazing ideas. You will succeed in those ideas! You will prove to yourself and others that there was a method behind all the jobs that you had over the years!

Love you.

~Your Admirer

#11

I affirm my happiness.
I affirm my happiness.
I affirm my happiness.

5/12/17

"Say in your head,
I affirm my happiness."

Hey Boo!

You're on my mind. I was thinking about your depressed states and realized that during those states it can feel impossible to do anything that can heal you in the moment. To make it easier on yourself, one simple thing you can do is affirm your happiness even during the present depressed state. Say in your head, I affirm my happiness. If you can, repeat it as many times as you can. And even better, you can push yourself to write it down a few times. This affirmation can help you climb out of this state and/or give you more hope that you will get through it. I affirm your happiness.

Kisses and hugs,

You know who :)

Letters to My Bipolar Self

Write notes or your own letter:

#12

Feeling Good

5/18/17

"So the answers are already within you."

My love!! Hey girl, hey!!

From what you have expressed to me, you've been feeling good! So I want you to capture this moment to view at another time when that feeling might be compromised. One thing that I think contributed to you feeling this way is when you were reminded to affirm your happiness. And remember, you were reminded because YOU told someone else to affirm their wellness. That's right, YOU did that. So the answers are already within you. Good job at giving the advice and in recognizing that you needed to flip that advice toward yourself. And even better, you did well in taking action by affirming your happiness in your mind during depressive or anxious states and by also putting a Post-it on your door that reads, "I affirm my happiness." Keep rising! You're doing so well and I am very proud of you!

Love you to pieces! xoxo

~You know who <wink>

Letters to My Bipolar Self

Write notes or your own letter:

#13

Feeling Stuck

7/6/17

"...don't get stuck in feeling
stuck."

My Sweet Drizzle,

You were feeling stuck and started having irrational thoughts that you need to make big decisions and moves that aren't possible yet. You were very frustrated. When you feel this way, you have to use the moments to fuel and motivate you to come up with creative ideas on what you can do in the moment. For example, if you are in a rut about feeling stuck financially, you can be creative on what you can do currently to increase your finances.

When you start to feel stuck or frustrated about your current situation, don't get *stuck* in feeling stuck. Be empowered when feeling stuck. Use those feelings to motivate you, not deteriorate you.

Unstuckingly,

Your Vegan Apple Pie

Letters to My Bipolar Self

Write notes or your own letter:

#14

Describing Your Symptoms

7/7/17

"...this is another affirmation showing that you are not alone."

Hey my love,

Trust yourself when you explain how your symptoms feel. When you feel like you are drowning (figuratively)...

When you feel stuck...

When you feel confined...

When you feel like your blood is boiling...

When you feel like you can't explain how you feel but feel as if you are in a pre-depression stage...

Looking back at how you would describe your feelings, you tend to laugh because you think it sounds silly. But your therapist made such a good point! First, she mentioned not to laugh at yourself because it makes sense. Then, she also mentioned that she hears those descriptions often, so it's not as uncommon as you might feel. I know that was quite shocking but this is another affirmation showing that you are not alone. The next time you ponder to describe how you are feeling and come up with your own terminology, validate it.

Love you,
mwen menm*

*English translation: Myself

Letters to My Bipolar Self

Write notes or your own letter:

#15

The Four Agreements

7/7/17

"Whenever you follow these agreements, you are contributing to your mental wellness."

Hey again|

Geez- I seem to have a lot to tell you today (or rather tonight because it's 2am and I'm still up, energized) One of our favorite books is *The Four Agreements*[1] by Don Miguel Ruiz and I just love how it talks about having four agreements with ourselves to help us be the best we can be. The four agreements are as follows:

1. Don't take anything personally.
2. Be impeccable with your word.
3. Do your best.
4. Don't make assumptions.

These agreements have drastically changed the way you think. No matter how much time has passed since you read the book, you constantly think about these agreements. Doing the opposite of these agreements, aggravates your mental health symptoms and contributes to your mental health issues. Whenever you follow these agreements, you are contributing to your mental wellness. Keep these agreements in mind as a tool toward bettering your mental health.

Yours forever,

G. L.

[1] Don Miguel Ruiz (2011)

Letters to My Bipolar Self

Write notes or your own letter:

#16

Piece by Piece

7/8/17

"Cherish each piece as they come little by little."

Hey!

Sometimes things come together piece by piece. Sometimes small pieces at a time. Hold on to each and every piece. Cherish each piece as they come little by little. Don't get consumed by the fact that you found a tiny little piece and that it will take forever to get anywhere. That's okay because a whole bunch of tiny little pieces can still be put together into one big piece, even if it takes longer.

It's all coming together.

Your Peacemaker

Letters to My Bipolar Self

Write notes or your own letter:

#17

You Have Bipolar

7/11/17

"You are not bipolar;
you just have bipolar."

Letters to My Bipolar Self

Hey my love,

Your diagnosis was on my mind and I wanted to share with you how I perceive it.

You are not bipolar; you just have bipolar.

Bipolar is just something you have. If bipolar was who you were, you wouldn't have so many other great qualities. You are made up of so many more beautiful pieces. When speaking about having bipolar, avoid saying that you "are" bipolar.

If it slips out just out of habit, just correct yourself.

Say it to yourself now: I am not bipolar.

Yours forever,

IANB

Letters to My Bipolar Self

Write notes or your own letter:

#18

Uplifting Your Mood

7/22/17

"Honor and validate your
feelings and efforts
when you catch it."

Hey Sweetie,

You were on my mind and I thought of a good analogy when it comes to the recent mood drop that you experienced.

Your mood can drop in a matter of seconds and can easily reach rock bottom as fast as a penny can reach the ground from the 21st floor. You can make a fast decision as it drops by running to one of the lower floors and catching it before it reaches the ground. It is really challenging to do since it's going at 50mph, but I know you can do it! You also have to use time to heal fully from your dropped mood. Even if you catch it from the 7th floor, it can take time to get it up the stairs back to your original mood. Honor and validate your feelings and efforts when you catch it. If you don't see any improvement, go up one step at a time, one floor at a time and then allow time to help you get back up there! I promise how you feel on the current floor you are on can change if you truly believe it can change. Believe even if you can't see or feel it, and you will be back on the 21st floor, if not higher!

Keep climbing high at your own pace!

Love you so much,

Your admirer

Letters to My Bipolar Self

Write notes or your own letter:

#19

Mental Breakdown #3

10/16/17

"Your hospitalization does
not mean that you are weak."

Alo*,

It's been a while since I wrote you a letter because you were very sick and were hospitalized for almost 3 weeks in August. I missed you so much and was in so much pain to see you in pain...in mental pain. I am beyond proud of you for how far you've come and how well you handled your pain. Despite your intense anxiety, despite dealing with awful side effects from several medications, and despite dealing with other symptoms all at once, you never gave up and kept pushing through. You would focus on mental wellness affirmations and would also keep your eyes on God. You are very courageous and very strong! Your mental strength is high, higher than you might realize. Your hospitalization does not mean that you are weak. It's HOW you handle your hospitalization that measures your mental strength. And you handled it really well. Keep that in mind when your symptoms sneak up on you. Keep up the good work and keep striving. I know you are still in recovery so do your best to listen to your body.

I know you can do it! I love you so much.

~Your #1 Proud Supporter

*English translation: Hello

Letters to My Bipolar Self

Write notes or your own letter:

#20

Overcoming This Depressive State

12/8/17

"Don't let your depression
cripple you;
let it empower you."

Hey love,

The last few weeks have been challenging for you with all the depressive symptoms you've been having. The symptoms really drain your energy, making it almost impossible to do ANYTHING. I don't have a perfect solution to help you overcome this but I do have a few suggestions. First off, it's a good thing you started reading some of the other letters that have helped in boosting your mood and making you feel more hopeful in overcoming this state especially since you overcame it before.

Keep praying and asking God for guidance and wisdom to get through these symptoms. Make meditation a part of your routine. There's been a lot of success stories on meditation and mental health but you have to be consistent. Try to meditate once a day. Don't give up. Keep pushing and pushing and pushing and pushing through your low energy, feelings of sadness, etc. Don't let your depression cripple you; let it empower you.

Claim your energy back! You are going to overcome this depressive state. I really believe in you and know you are strong enough to push it aside!

I love you.

~Your #1 Fan

Letters to My Bipolar Self

Write notes or your own letter:

#21

Feeling Lost and Unmotivated

12/20/17

"It cannot stay foggy
forever."

My dearest love,

You are going through a challenging time of feeling lost and unmotivated. Some of it has to do with the depressive states that you've been having. Your depression is up and down: some weeks are better than others. There's no perfect formula that I can give you to overcome this stage but what I will say is to keep pushing through even if everything seems so foggy. It cannot stay foggy forever. You will reach the other side of the fog and get your motivation back. What you are feeling is just a season. Accept the season but also find hope within yourself that things will change for the better. Keep your focus on God so that he can deliver you from this season. I believe in you and know that you are strong enough to fight and win!

I'm rooting for you!

Love,

Your admirer

Letters to My Bipolar Self

Write notes or your own letter:

#22

Balancing Mental Strength

2/3/18

"In some ways your strength blinds you from the intensity of your symptoms."

Hey my love,

One thing I admire about you is how strong you are mentally. You've built a significant amount of mental strength over the years. No matter what symptoms you are experiencing, you conquer and conquer and conquer! You keep pushing through.

While it is great that you have such mental strength, you have to balance your strength. In some ways your strength blinds you from the intensity of your symptoms. You push yourself so far that you don't realize how much you are going through. One example is the trauma you experienced within the last year. You had two mental breakdowns in under a year. The first one you fought through it and avoided hospitalization. The second one you ended up in 2 different hospitals for a total of 3 weeks, then you had to recover, then you were having constant side effects from so many different medications they were putting you on and then within 2 months you were planning a major event. That's a lot to go through but with your strength you fought through it. It's good that you used your mental strength but you didn't give yourself time to accept how much you were going through. It's only after a few people mentioned that you've been through a lot that you started to realize it. And now you realize it the most because you've been suffering from severe depression. You don't know the full cause but one reason is definitely your body and mind catching up from all that you went through mentally. What's important is that you are recognizing that your strength can actually hinder you from fully recovering. Keep up with conquering your mental health and building your mental strength but balance your strength. Use your strength to push through any symptoms while also recognizing the intensity of your symptoms and the affect those symptoms have on you. Recognizing that your symptoms are intense or extremely painful doesn't mean that you are weak: it actually shows strength.

Keep showing off and building that amazing mental strength of yours.

Stay strong,

Your Personal Trainer

#23

Feeling Like You're Not Enough

2/28/18

"You even told yourself that
you are not enough."

My Everything,

Today was a HUGE success in celebrating your sister's birthday. You ended the day with an amazing Broadway production of one of her favorite movies, *Frozen*! The cast and production staff were incredibly talented!!!! You were so blown away by every aspect of the show. Despite such an amazing experience, you started feeling down. Those feelings turned into you not feeling good about yourself and not feeling that you are enough. You started to question what you were doing after seeing all the great things that the people in the show were doing. You even told yourself that you are not enough. Well I'm here to tell you the harsh reality: You ARE enough. You are more than enough. Telling yourself that you are not enough makes it even harder for you to be your best potential self. Don't bring yourself down because you are not where you would like to be. Use those feelings as motivation to work more and be productive. I believe in all your dreams and aspirations! It can be done and it can be done by YOU. Don't be afraid of the steps you need to take to get there. Just take whatever steps that you can. Be patient and kind to yourself during the process. And remember, you ARE enough.

Love you to pieces,

Your Shining Light

Letters to My Bipolar Self

Write notes or your own letter:

#24

Fears of Another Breakdown

3/5/18

"Don't be afraid...
be prepared."

My Dearest Warrior,

Sometimes you have fears of having another breakdown. Don't be afraid...be prepared. Of course you can affirm that it won't happen, but if for any reason it does, you are prepared and strong enough to handle it. Remember this the next time your mind tricks you into worrying that another one is coming again.

Stay encouraged,

G.

Letters to My Bipolar Self

Write notes or your own letter:

#25

Experiencing Some Symptoms

4/14/18

"These moments are a good reminder to practice more rituals daily..."

Hey my love,

I know you have been having some anxiety and irritability lately and you are not even sure where it is coming from. Sometimes it is simply coming from your diagnosis. It is part of having bipolar disorder. I am proud of you for recognizing the symptoms early on and taking some initiative to manage them. These moments are a good reminder to practice more rituals daily, such as meditation and drinking tea at night.

I am really glad that you decided to go on that walk to the pier even though you were starting to get comfortable at home. For you, nature has miraculous healing properties when it comes to your mental health and you took such a beneficial step by going on that walk.

Kenbe la*,

Your Healer

*English translation: Hang in there

Letters to My Bipolar Self

Write notes or your own letter:

#26

Good Things About Being Hospitalized

5/5/18

"I'm not sure if you would have survived without them."

To the one who completes me,

Today I'm writing to you to help you recognize that there is actually some good that has come out of all your hospitalizations in the psychiatric unit. I made a list that I am going to share with you.

Good Things About Being Hospitalized:

1. You were reminded of the amazing support system that you have from friends and family. Your dad visited you every day, TWO times a day. Your mom came every day after work. Your sister traveled from far to see you often and bring you your favorite foods and activities to keep you busy. Other family members came to visit you or called to check up on you. Your friends made time to visit you even though they have never seen you in that state. I'm not sure if you would have survived without them. I know you are FOREVER grateful for such love and support.

2. From your first hospitalization, it showed you what can transpire from your mind and body when you are not doing well mentally or don't seek the help that you need beforehand.

3. You are more motivated to take good care of yourself mentally to avoid other hospitalizations.

4. You appreciate the small things more. On the psychiatric unit, you are trapped inside, depending

on the facility, and the windows are covered so you can't really see outside or go outside. Having the freedom to see trees and grass or go for a stroll is such a beautiful thing that can be taken for granted.

5. You are reminded to have more humility because it can happen to anyone and while you are on the unit you don't look like your best self.

6. You recognize that you are stronger than you think. Everything that you go through right before being hospitalized and during your hospital stay is a lot. You are able to fight and push through, while also uplifting yourself. After a hospital stay, you feel like a survivor.

You are a survivor! You have survived three hospitalizations. That number might seem small but the number to represent the intensity of your symptoms is really high during each hospital stay. And it takes you six months to a year to fully recover after each stay. So, let me emphasize that YOU ARE A SURVIVOR!

Your loving partner,

#27

Feeling at Peace

5/6/18

"...you are accepting where you are while looking forward to where you are going."

Hey Honey!

Someone's been feeling at peace! I'm so happy for you! I especially love that you are at peace not because everything is going right or going your way, but because you are accepting where you are while looking forward to where you are going. May your journey lead you to peace, peace, and more peace.

Namaste,

Your Peaceful Friend

Write notes or your own letter:

#28

How Long Will "Feeling Good" Last?

5/19/2018

"...you are more than
equipped to fight it and win!"

My greatest love! Hey!

I'm so happy to see that you've been feeling good. You haven't felt this good in a while with two mental breakdowns months apart and recovering from your last one. I know there's one question on your mind: how long will this last? I don't think anyone has the answer but focus on embracing and enjoying this moment. Be persistent in how you are caring for yourself. And most importantly, keep being mentally self-aware of your emotions and keep your eye out for any little symptom. All we can do is hope that this feeling lasts forever without any major symptoms. But just know that IF *knocks on wood* your symptoms come back to haunt you, you are more than equipped to fight it and win! So don't worry about your symptoms making an appearance, focus on feeling good and work on making it last!

Love ya,

Your Bestie

Write notes or your own letter:

#29

Try Again and Again

5/24/18

"When you do not succeed,
it does not mean
that you failed."

My beloved Glenda,

I'm going to keep this short and to the point.

Even when you don't succeed when trying to reach your goals, keep trying. Don't give up. Take time to focus on what you can learn or do differently going forward when you do not succeed in the moment. When you do not succeed, it does not mean that you failed. It just means that you need to be redirected toward a different path to reach the success that you desire.

Wishing you greater success than you can imagine,

Write notes or your own letter:

#30

Pace Yourself

5/25/18

"Any little step you take is
still a good thing."

My achiever,

When you feel like there are too many steps, pace yourself. Any little step you take is still a good thing. Even if you don't see results right away, acknowledge that you are taking steps toward your goal. The fact that you are taking the time to do even the smallest steps shows that you are committed to achieving what you want and setting yourself up for success. AND you are sending signals out there to the Universe when you take those steps (big or small).

Keep stepping toward success.

Sending you all my love,

Gee L.

Write notes or your own letter:

#31

Breaking Point

5/28/18

"It's not a good place to be in, but it has some good benefits."

My sweet love,

You have issues with oversleeping. You thought it was part of your depression but your therapist feels it's something physical. I agree with her. You've gotten testing done but need to do more testing. In the meantime, you feel like you are fed up with this sleeping pattern. It's affecting a lot of things. It's not a good place to be in, but it has some good benefits.

Being in this space pushes and motivates you more to get better and work on it in the best way possible until you find out what is really wrong. Take advantage of this place. I already see you making some changes like limiting your screen time before bed and going to bed earlier. You're doing good so far. It's a good start. It might not cure it, but it will definitely give you the opportunity to live better with it. I'm seeing the good in your not so good place. Look at it another way to see it too.

Best wishes,

Your Sweetheart

Write notes or your own letter:

#32

How To Practice Self-Reflection

6/2/18

"It's really magical and miraculous when that happens."

Hey love|

I noticed that self-reflection is very crucial for your mental health and for managing your symptoms. When you are consistently reflecting on your mental state you can notice symptoms sooner and stop certain symptoms from escalating into something bigger. It also gives you the time to learn more about yourself and make healthy decisions for your mental well-being. Sometimes, you need to set aside a specific time to analyze your thoughts and to think deeply about anything that is on your mind. Other times, you don't have to do much to analyze. All you need to do is be by yourself in a peaceful and therapeutic place while allowing your thoughts to just be. You will realize over time that you are self-reflecting quite naturally and might even come up with solutions to problems that were on your mind. It's really magical and miraculous when that happens. I notice that you experience this when you go by yourself to a body of water near a pier or a beach. You go to an area where you are not easily distracted by anyone else, get lost gazing into the water, and then let your thoughts flow. That's an example of self-reflection. Keep going by the water on a consistent basis and don't give it too much thought on self-reflecting. Let nature do the work to flow in and out of you.

Namaste,

Your Peace Warrior

Write notes or your own letter:

#33

Your Mind is Your Friend

6/2/18

"Learn to love your mind
even through those times..."

Hello again!!

Missed me?

With bipolar there are times where your mind seems to be attacking you. That doesn't mean that your mind can't be good for you. Your mind can actually be your friend. There are so many reasons why your mind attacks you.

1. When you treat your mind badly, it eventually has a defensive mechanism where it fights back to make you aware of how badly you are treating it.

2. The mind gets so sick when your symptoms get really bad that it becomes unbearable for the mind. The mind then lashes out at you in the form of chest pains or uncontrollable thoughts because you are the one closest by for the mind to react to. Think of the analogy of a woman giving birth and screams at her husband who is next to her or slaps her best friend who is telling her to push. Society is okay when such reactions occur, but when our mind is in pain and acts out on the body through hallucinations, for example, people judge and see the mind as toxic. Or people judge those who are having those reactions and acting a certain way.

Recognize and accept whatever reactions you are experiencing, but don't judge your mind for causing those reactions. Learn to love your mind even through those times and over time you will see how amazing your mind can be. You and your mind can still be friends despite the moments when it attacks.

Be enlightened,

Your Mind's Assistant

#34

Suicidal Thoughts

6/6/18

"Sometimes you have survivor's guilt..."

My precious Glenda,

Sadly, you used to have many suicidal thoughts. They were passive thoughts since you never had any intention or plan to act on them. It is still scary to think that you even considered and fantasized about suicide. I am so proud of you that you have been healed and no longer have those thoughts.

Every time you hear of someone committing suicide, it brings you back to a time when you had such ideations. This happened yesterday when you heard that Kate Spade passed away by committing suicide. Sometimes you have survivor's guilt, but just know you survived to spare your loved ones the hurt. You also get to live to tell your story and save other lives.

With purest love, kisses and hugs,

Your Sunshine

Write notes or your own letter:

#35

You Looked Beautiful

6/12/18

"Let this be evidence that you
ARE beautiful on the outside
(and on the inside too)"

Hey Beautiful!

You looked so pretty today, Glenda! It wasn't a special occasion or a fancy outfit. You were wearing casual clothes with your hair pulled back and practically no makeup. Even with minimal effort, you still looked beautiful! I'm saying this to you to help you through those days that you don't feel beautiful; those days that you don't like what you are wearing; those days that you are not happy with your perfectly imperfect body; those days that you wish you had different features; those days that you don't love yourself because of the way that you look; those days that your mood is low because of how you feel about how you look. Let this be evidence that you ARE beautiful on the outside (and inside)! It's ok that you have days that you don't look your best, but that doesn't stop your beauty from shining on the outside.

Love you Beautiful,

Your favorite mirror

Write notes or your own letter:

#36

"Mentally ill"

6/13/18

"...I don't label you as mentally ill."

Letters to My Bipolar Self

Hey my love,

I wanted you to keep in mind some affirmations based on who you are. Even though you have bipolar, I don't label you as mentally ill. There is a lot of stigma around the terms mentally ill and mental illness. You don't have to associate yourself with those terms. Since you are not mentally ill, below is a list of who you are. Use this list to serve as a reminder of who you really are.

You are a woman.
You are Haitian.
You are beautiful.
You are smart.
You are creative.
You are passionate.
You are a musician.
You are a writer.
You are a survivor.
You are inspirational.
You are mentally strong.

And most importantly, you are loved...by me.

I love you,

G.

Write notes or your own letter

#37

Freedom Because of Bipolar

6/13/18

"Look at all that bipolar has done for you."

To the one who completes me,

Believe it or not, your first mental breakdown and your bipolar diagnosis gave you freedom. Yup, you read right. Freedom. You have changed and you are now more outspoken and passionate. Before your breakdown, you hid your true self with your symptoms for so long that you could not even own up to it for your own self. Once you owned it and admitted that you needed help, you were able to be more open overall.

You also have to remember that you are a survivor. You survived your first mental breakdown (and the others that came after). That gave you more confidence in yourself for getting through something you did not know you were even capable of getting through. After your breakdown, you felt like you were given a second chance at life, so you took that chance and ran! That's really great! You are more energetic, more bold, and more expressive. Look at all that bipolar has done for you.

Who said bipolar was so bad?

Unconditionally yours,

Your Survivor Manual

Write notes or your own letter:

#38

Happiness

6/18/18

"I am happy. I deserve to
show my happiness."

Hey Sunshine,

Why do you sometimes feel shy or uncomfortable showing people or expressing your happiness?

Maybe it stems from a time when you didn't allow yourself to show your happiness.

Maybe it stems from a time when you didn't think you were worthy of experiencing happiness.

Maybe it stems from a time when you didn't love yourself and therefore weren't happy.

Whatever the reason, just know that you are not that same person from your past. You were very unhealthy mentally and now you are so much stronger mentally! You found ways to love yourself and you deserve to feel and express your happiness! Don't be shy about it. Own it and admit it to yourself. Take the time right now and repeat, "I am happy. I deserve to show my happiness." Maybe even make it your current affirmation!

Love,

Your Happy Twin

Write notes or your own letter:

#39

Defining Trauma

7/4/18

"Trauma is defined by the
individual experiencing it."

Hey My Love,

Let's discuss the true definition of trauma. Trauma is defined by the individual experiencing it. People shouldn't tell someone what should or shouldn't be traumatic to them. That's how people remain hurt with mental issues for years.

For example, if a cop hears gunshots every day and someone who never hears gunshots hears it for the first time, that person can be traumatized while the cop might not be in the moment. That doesn't make the person's trauma any less authentic.

You have to accept what you call trauma and not bring yourself down for having traumatic experiences that society or anyone else might not think is traumatic. What's important is that you recognize what is traumatic to you so that you can work on it. I respect what you consider traumatic and I am here for you if you ever need anything.

Love,

Gee Lenz

Write notes or your own letter:

#40

Use Your Toolbox

7/4/18

"Use your toolbox, but sometimes you might need to go to the hardware store..."

Letters to My Bipolar Self

Bonswa*,

Your therapist talks about using your toolbox and adding tools to help you with your symptoms. She also mentions that sometimes some tools might not work in the moment and that's ok.

Use your toolbox, but sometimes you might need to go to the hardware store and get other screws or bolts or maybe even a whole other tool. Sometimes you might only need a piece from the hardware store to attach to a tool in your current toolbox. Other times you might need to go from store to store until you find what you need.

Any time you overcome a symptom or mental health state, you have to analyze to see what you did right and what you learned from it. You can always learn something and that something can be added to your toolbox. You already tend to do this both consciously and unconsciously. It's ok to not always have all the tools you need. Just be creative with what you have and then go from store to store until you find what fits.

Keep using tools to build,

G the Builder

*English translation: Good Afternoon

Write notes or your own letter:

#41

Your First Therapist

7/5/18

"Sometimes therapy doesn't
work out because we don't
allow it to."

Hey There!

I was looking back at your first therapy sessions and realized that the thought of therapy can be a scary thing. Some people have never tried it because of the stigma and negative perceptions of therapy. Some people tried it but had a bad experience.

I'm sure you would agree that therapy is one of the best things that has happened to you! I am a huge advocate for therapy and recommend it to anyone and everyone. I know as an advocate, you do the same. The interesting part is you didn't always feel this way. You had so many misconceptions and fears about therapy.

You finally went after your first breakdown and hospitalization. You honestly only went because you wanted to get better and knew that therapy was one of the ways to get better. When you started going, you were very closed. You had a wall up. You didn't hate it but you didn't love it. Your emotions were so obvious that your first therapist had to ask if therapy was what you even wanted! You told her that you felt like it's something that you needed, so pretty much saying that you had no choice. After that, you started opening up and telling her your reservations about therapy. She answered all your questions and debunked any myths that you believed. Fast forward a few sessions and you actually started loving it!!!! She is literally one of the best therapists that you ever

163

had. If you didn't stay longer, you would have thought that therapy wasn't for you or would have labeled her as a bad therapist when she wasn't even the issue. Sometimes therapy doesn't work out because we don't allow it to. We don't allow ourselves to open up and see the benefit in it. It is beautiful to see that you allowed yourself to open up to therapy and now you continue to see the amazing benefits in it.

Keep on thriving with your therapy journey and continue to be an example to those in therapy or seeking therapy.

Love,

Your Advocate

#42

A Message From a Cough Drop

7/25/18

"...remind yourself to not give up on yourself."

Hey My Sick One,

You have been battling a cold, so you have been taking steps to get better. One thing that you have been doing is eating cough drops. Of course the Universe finds ways to communicate with you about mental health even when you are sick with a cold. The cough drop wrapper had motivating phrases on them. Two of the phrases on the wrapper stood out to you.

"You've survived tougher."

"Don't give up on yourself."

While those statements are relevant if you are sick with a cold or the flu, you recognized that they can also be very pertinent to your journey with bipolar. Whenever you have a symptom that is intense or seems impossible to overcome, remind yourself to not give up on yourself. Remind yourself that you have survived tougher. You are worth the fight.

Your Fellow Fighter,

The **M**atriarch **M**agical **A**dmirable (MMA) Fighter

Write notes or your own letter:

#43

Don't Be Hard on Yourself

7/28/18

"You chose to take care of
yourself first."

Hey you|

I'm so happy to see that you are still feeling well mentally! There is one thing that is bothering you a little though: not having a job.

Yes, you've been applying and yes, you are picky with what you are looking for and yes, you could be doing more but it's okay that you haven't found one yet. Don't beat yourself up too much.

First, be grateful that you have overwhelming support from your parents and your sister. Your basic needs are met, thanks to them. That's most important right now: you have a home, a bed to sleep in, clothes, and food.

The next thing I want you to keep in mind is that I want you to remember that almost this time last year you were in the hospital for weeks! And after you got out, it took you months to fully recover which means that for a while you did not feel well enough to work. It's not until a few months ago that you started feeling like you were able to work again. So I know it feels like almost a year since you haven't worked but most of that year you were focusing on your mental health and focusing on recovery. That is brave!! You chose to take care of yourself first. Who knows where you would be if you didn't recover. So be proud of yourself for taking your mental wellness seriously. I know that you had a major setback for doing so, but that's ok! Just remind yourself of all that you've been through a year ago and how far you have come.

I love you and I am very proud of you. Keep applying to those jobs and pray, pray, and pray! You will find one soon.

Love,

Your Sweetheart

#44

You're Happy

8/10/18

"You deserve to be happy just like anyone else."

The Happy One with Bipolar,

Just because you have bipolar, doesn't mean you can't be happy or will never experience happiness. Look at how you've been feeling lately. It's challenging for you to admit and accept the happiness you have been experiencing, so I challenge you to accept and embrace it. You deserve to be happy just like anyone else. Don't let any mental health condition tell you otherwise! And don't let your mind tell you that it won't last or that it's going to end soon since you have bipolar. Yes, anything is possible and you have to be aware of any triggers or symptoms, but that doesn't mean you can't experience lasting happiness. Whatever you believe to be true, will be true.

I wish you continuous happiness!!

Love,

Your Happiness Supporter

Write notes or your own letter:

#45

Focus on the Dolphins, Not the Sharks

8/18/18

"...don't get trapped into the delusion that you see a dolphin coming from far away when it's really a shark."

Hey pretty girl!

Yes, yes - I know. You are not feeling very pretty right now. That's why I need to remind you that you are pretty and you should love everything that you consider a flaw.

I realized that you just started feeling a little down, so I wanted to write you this letter. I know you don't know the full reason why your mood is this way and I know it's not just about your low confidence about your beauty.

The good thing is you noticed it very early on. Pay attention to moments like this when you begin to feel down; when your mood is about to shift. Once you notice it, you may not be able to completely remove the emotions that you are feeling, but stop it from accelerating down. This is a skill within itself, so don't be discouraged if it doesn't happen when you are first trying it. I'm very proud of you for being in this funky mood, but still pushing to stop yourself from getting worse. You have been good at recognizing your symptoms and being proactive at maintaining your mood to avoid it from dropping super low. Just know that moods and emotions come and go. Don't let ANY negative emotions stop you from staying afloat. Based off of your past and your instincts, you have dived into deep waters that led you to try to swim amongst the sharks of your emotions. Lately, you have been swimming with the dolphins of your emotions, where you are playful and fearless, but don't get trapped into the delusion that you see a dolphin coming from far away when it's really a shark. Whenever a shark tries to approach you, keep your eyes and your focus on the dolphins. You can't stop sharks from approaching, but you can stop them from drowning you.

Focus on the dolphins.
Focus on recognizing when your emotions are diving down as it is happening.
Focus on surfing the waves as they come.
Focus on flowing just like the ocean's water.
Focus on your strength to stay afloat.

Keep on flowing.

Love,

You know who :)

#46

Float Until You Reach the Sand

8/18/18

"You almost
feel your throat closing."

Hey again!

So I know you are starting to feel better, but I just wanted to recap how you were feeling after my letter while thinking about your low mood.

So, a lot of things combined led you to your room to do damage control to stay afloat and prevent yourself from sinking. You almost felt the tears coming out. You almost feel your throat closing. You almost felt your chest sinking, BUT above all you decided to F-L-O-A-T. You acknowledged what you were feeling, but floated toward water that wasn't as deep; toward water that you could comfortably stand in; toward water that is low enough where you can manage your emotions. You told yourself that you would survive.

You will get through it. You will love yourself better. You will end up on the sand, laying down relaxing. You just have to keep floating until you reach there. Don't allow yourself to keep drowning and sinking deeper, especially since I know that once you sink it becomes a lot more challenging to float. It becomes a lot more challenging to get back to the sand. It also takes a lot longer as well. It's better to start now and focus on continuously floating toward the sand.

Do this visual exercise:

Take a moment now to take 3 deep breaths. Imagine

that you are floating; floating in the strong currents while floating toward the sand. You've made it. You are on the sand now lying on a beautiful beach towel with sunglasses on protecting you from the dangerous negative rays.

Shine bright,

Your Sunshine

#47

Feeling More Motivated and Energized

9/9/18

"I also think all those affirmations you have spoken over your life are beginning to manifest."

Hey Sweetie!

The other day you had a moment...an epiphany. You felt like the person you were before your first mental breakdown. It was a good feeling! You still had mental health symptoms back then that were undiagnosed and that you were in denial about, but your most intense symptoms occurred during and after your first breakdown. Ever since that breakdown, certain things have not been the same. Your energy levels have decreased and you lost some of your motivation, but the other day you felt motivated again. You felt more energized and fully able to enjoy life. Don't get me wrong, you became a new and better person after your first breakdown when you changed your life, but you also lost something as well. You now have less energy, more sluggishness, and more fatigue. It keeps getting worse and worse as the years go by.

It's miraculous how you felt the other day and how you continue to feel. I also think all those affirmations you have spoken over your life are beginning to manifest. You didn't give up on those affirmations, even when it felt impossible.

There are many possible reasons as to why you felt more motivated and energized just like you used to feel. You finally admitted your calling for social work and you also finally accepted that you belong in another city. Finally, you have a plan to accomplish both: go to graduate school for social work in another city than the one you are currently living in. When you answer the call to fulfill your purpose, everything starts to align piece by piece. Even if you don't have all the pieces to complete the puzzle, you will start to feel whole. You have enough pieces to see the concept of the puzzle picture. Continue to align all the pieces that you have until the picture is completed.

One piece at a time,

Your Puzzle Maker

#48

Being Happy Despite Some Imperfections

9/12/18

"Things haven't been perfect,
but you are happy."

Hey There happy camper!

Wow! You are finally at a place where you feel happy despite some flaws and imperfections! Please take a moment (right now) to really soak in this victory and congratulate yourself for reaching this milestone. This is huge...bigger than you may realize! I know you are not sure how you reached this milestone, but remain present and grateful in the moment. Keep holding on to your excitement of the future. Even though you are still experiencing some issues at the moment, you still feel happy. Even though you are going through some anxiety and some other stuff, you still feel happy. Things haven't been perfect, but you are happy.

Keep up with your happiness.
Your happiness makes me happy.

I am proud of you,

~Your Proud Friend

Write notes or your own letter:

#49

The Benefits of Pushing Through

9/21/18

"Your symptoms don't have
to be permanent."

Letters to My Bipolar Self

Alo*,

I wanted to share with you the benefits you recently experienced because you pushed through.

There are rewards for pushing through and getting through symptoms. Your symptoms don't have to be permanent. It all starts with your mentality to remind yourself of that. You were having anxiety recently, but you kept getting yourself through it each time it happened. You did not allow yourself to obsess over it. At times, the anxiety felt like it would never go away and that you would just have to adjust to it being there all the time. Now, you realize, that is not true. Not only do you not have anxiety, but you actually feel really good! Your breathing is back to normal; your chest feels refreshed; your chest does not feel so heavy and weighed down. This goes to show you that your symptoms can only be permanent and consistent if you give them permission to be.

Pushing through your anxiety really helped you overcome it. Part of pushing through is accepting: accepting where you are at the current stage. You also have to refrain from judging yourself for feeling a certain way. You have to tell yourself that you are feeling *xyz* and that it's okay to have that feeling. Your mind and your brain needs reassurance that it's okay and it will be okay.

You are okay, even if your anxiety comes back.

Keep pushing,

Your Favorite Motivator

*English translation: Hello

#50

Growth Is Beautiful

11/5/18

"I am proud of you for being able to do this..."

My dearest love,

You are doing so well...actually extremely well! It is beautiful to see how much you have grown and how mentally strong you are becoming. I especially see your strength by the way you handle your symptoms and by the way you cope with negative mentalities that you may have.

One perfect example was the incident that happened at church yesterday. When you reached church, there weren't any more seats. One of the ushers told you to stand downstairs because someone will be adding more chairs. There were a lot of people waiting for chairs and you wanted to make sure you got a seat. As they started adding seats, you quickly went to sit, but one of the ushers told you not to sit yet because they wanted to finish setting up. You went back on the side to wait, but then other people still continued to sit. When you saw that, you decided to disregard the usher and just go back to sit. Again, the usher told you specifically that you can't sit yet.

This moment led you to being extremely frustrated. You started thinking about how part of the problem is the overpopulation of New York City and how everything you want to do turns into a hustle. You were frustrated to the point that you were on the verge of tears and it took some time for you to feel better. One thing that you did do in the moment, is that you turned your frustration into a moment of reflection by focusing on the things you would want in another city that you move to instead of focusing on what you don't want while living in NYC. You also comforted yourself in the moment with loving words and by finding ways to distract yourself. Instead of breaking down crying, you were able to tell yourself to eat a mint to distract your mind and keep yourself calm. By the end of the service, you were back to your perky self.

This moment shows that you allowed yourself to have these negative emotions without judging yourself while finding ways to comfort yourself. I am proud of you for being able to do this because years ago, you would have beat yourself up for getting frustrated and you would have stayed frustrated for a longer period of time. Negative emotions are natural, but how you choose to handle them can be unnatural and unhealthy.

Naturally,

Your G.

Letters to My Bipolar Self

Write notes or your own letter:

My Dearest Readers,

Thank you tremendously for reading my book. I hope it has touched your heart! There are no words to describe how your support makes me feel.

I would love to know what you thought of my book! Let me know your thoughts on any of my platforms below. Also, feel free to leave a review on Amazon.

Stay in touch!

www.risingfrombipolar.com
risingfrombipolar@gmail.com

With love,

Glenda

Author | Blogger | Mental Wellness Advocate